How to get strong FAST

By Jack F. Jordan

Dedication

To my best friend, Alex, who had too little time on this Planet to achieve his dreams.

Preface

Here's the deal. You considered lifting weights. You tried getting o
the treadmill and running a marathon, or even joining an MMA c
Boxing class. But you just didn't have it in you. You are not stron
enough. You are not making any progress.

Well guess what. I used to be you. In this book, you will learn how t
get strong FAST and overcome tough challenges in a much shorte
time than anyone else would have let on. If you get good enough wit
the stuff taught in this book, you will potentially reach superhuma
levels.

And that is a promise.

This book is based on one portion of the knowledge I have acquire
through my years of experience observing the same kinds of peopl
struggle with improving their strength. Too many fitness gurus requir
that you train for years without results. Going from zero to hero ca
be frustrating and this book will ease you into becoming a fitte
stronger individual within as little as three months.

If you follow the instructions in this book word for word, then by th
end of it you will be running further and doing more push-ups tha
you previously thought possible, among other things. Believe me,
went from being able to do three push-ups at most to doing a hundre
all within only two months.

What's even more astonishing is while I used to get tired after runnin
a couple of feet, I could run six miles in less than an hour withou
getting tired. I could do all of this simply because I discovered a fe
secrets. These are the secrets I will be sharing with you in this book.

I can tell you are up to the challenge. Read this book from end to en
and follow its teachings. A little commitment will go a long way.

Kind Regards, Jack F. Jordan

Contents

Check Your Diet Before Doing Anything Else

The first thing you need to do before any form of strength training is to get your diet in check. Are you out of shape or not? The BMI scale doesn't help much and is outdated. I prefer the waist to height measurement. Take a recording of your height and a measure of your waist, then find yourself on the chart.

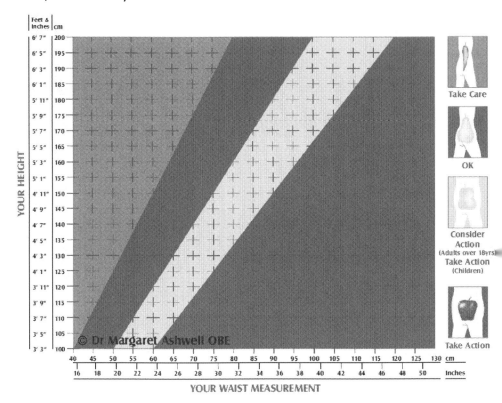

YOUR WAIST MEASUREMENT

If you are either under or overweight, consider changing your diet. You'll want to keep it balanced and consistent. The same advice applies if you are healthy according to the measure. But remember, It's just that. A measure attempting to classify your health. If in doubt, arrange for a physical check up with your doctor. For a more detailed guide to dietary hacks, stay on the lookout for my follow up books.

If you fear you are **overweight** or obese, start to control your portions.

Portion control is the key to battling obesity.

ere is a question I want you to answer: How many hours could you ɔ on a large bowl of cereal muesli?

e honest with yourself. Just look at the bowl.

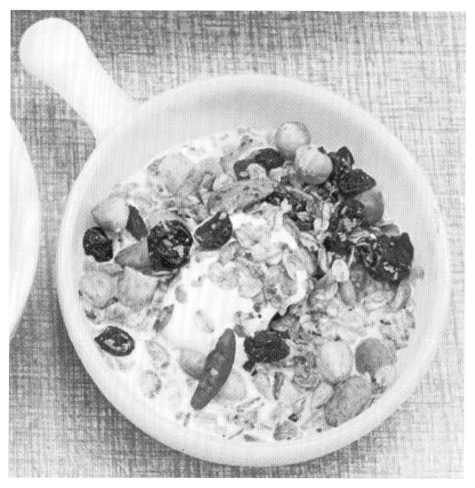

ɔw suppose I halve the bowl of cereals. You wake up at six thirty in e morning and eat the first half. Then as you are about to go out at ght, you eat the second half.

ɔw long do you think you could go now?

stonishingly, scientific studies have shown that smaller portions hich are spread out across the day keep you satisfied for longer. Even hen the total amount of food you eat decreases.

Not only that but people who are overweight tend to snack more Meaning that you cause the most damage to your health when you are not paying attention. That is why I typically discourage relentless snacking and prefer to eat food as part of a meal. The only snacks I eat are nuts and berries during breakfast or dinner.

Try controlling your portions. It will do wonders for your body.

Another thing to keep in mind is that you do not want to be eating right before you go to bed, or in the three hours before it. When you eat, your body experiences a glucose rush. Sleeping during this time will build up great levels of fat beneath the skin. This is in fact a technique used by Sumo wrestlers to put on fat.

In summary, Eat less food but more frequently. That is the key to losing weight.

Fasting, on the other hand, can be detrimental to your health. Many obese people who went on to lose weight experienced extreme loose skin as shown.

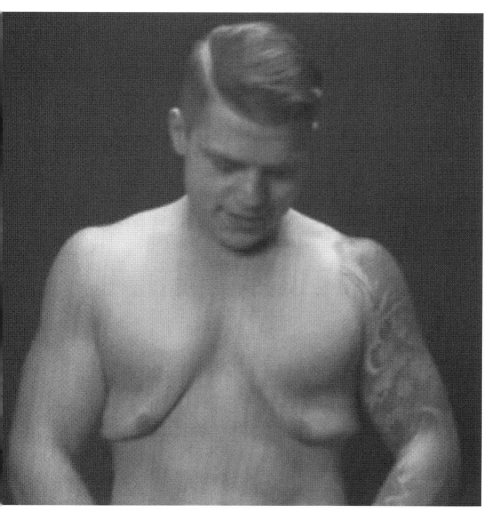

nis would not have happened if they had controlled their portions nd lost weight at a steady pace while at the same time getting ronger and developing muscle tissue, as covered in this book.

preading your food intake across the day allows you to digest food ore steadily and lose weight, as your desire for each meal lessens. nere is one last thing you must know if you are overweight. I like to all this the evil of all evils.

ugar.

pout fifty years ago, the average person would eat something sweet nce a week. You read that right. Once a week. It turns out that sugar raises your cholesterol and threatens you with heart disease. Not fat. Sixty percent of obese people gain weight because of their sugar intake, not their fat intake. Sugar forces your brain to release huge levels of dopamine, making it just as addictive as abusive drugs.

Too much Sugar will give you cancer.

Uncontrolled levels of cell growth cause cancer. Insulin is one of the hormones which regulates this. That is why eating a lot of sugar elevates your body's insulin levels and puts you at a greater risk of getting cancer.

I was friends with an obese woman who told me no matter how healthily she ate, she simple could not lose weight. That was before she told me that her diet consisted of seven Oranges a day, among other sweet fruits. The amount of sugar she was getting from supposedly healthy fruits was too much. I got her to eat vegetables and nuts instead. Although she was addicted to the sugar she had been getting, she stuck with my prescribed diet. Only a few weeks later she had lost twenty pounds. That is almost ten kilograms. Go pick up a ten-kilogram weight at the gym. Now imagine having to carry that around with you every single day of your life. Imagine the relief she experienced when she let go of those twenty pounds of fat.

Are you overweight? you can feel the same relief my friend felt simply by cutting down on your sugar intake. And while you are at it, read the rest of the book to become strong FAST!

If you feel **underweight**, then plan a regular diet of carbohydrates and proteins. When I started out I was 6'1'' and weighed 154lbs. I vowed to gain mass so that my ribs would not show. I got the results I needed after about three months of eating four large meals every day.

Eat your proteins and carbohydrates first, then your vegetables, and then drink water. You need to take in all the amino acids your body needs. Meat and Fish are perfect for this. Why? Because the animal hat the meat belonged to needed the same amino acids! Thus, the amino acids are present in their meat and ready for you to eat.

f you want to eat something other than meat and still get the right balance of amino acids, then mix different grains together. Rice and Beans together are the tried and tested age-old combination.

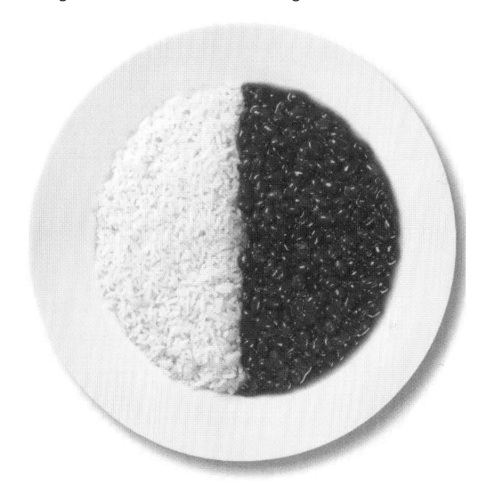

here are additional ways to gain weight. One of them is to eat and en sleep immediately afterwards. The rush of glucose to your blood used by eating food requires your body to start moving. When you eep, all this energy is forced to be stored as a layer of fat under the in. This is the same technique used by Sumo Wrestlers to gain mass and you can use it to gain weight that you will convert to muscle through strength training.

However, the best way to pull this off is to sleep, wake up before sunrise. Eat. Go back to Sleep. Then wake up in the morning. Eating before dinner does not give you the same benefits of weight gain. That is why you might want to consider changing your sleep schedule around, as covered in a later chapter.

Here is one final tip regardless of whether your goal is weight gain, loss, or maintenance: Stay hydrated. I was surprised to find that the recommended daily intake of water for a grown male is about 3.7 Litres. There used to be days that I would go without drinking any water, because I could not afford to spend too much money or bottles. That was until I bought myself a water filter like the one shown here.

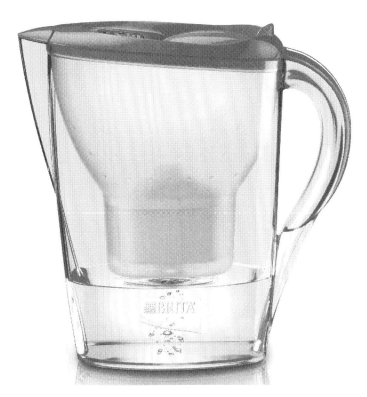

Run tap water through it and it will be drinkable. You have an endless supply of water in your kitchen. Put it to good use!

Here's the deal. This book is about getting strong FAST. As far as dietary gains are concerned a chocolate or fruit shake is the perfect recovery tool. I do not recommend protein shakes because the protein powder must be weighed with respect to the other nutrients you consume throughout the day. Most people like to consume protein shakes an hour before exercise. I believe that this is not beneficial since it can affect your performance depending on the type of strength you will need to display. To create a chocolate or fruit shake, simply mix your raw ingredients with milk or water in a blender. Then consume this after training, as a recovery option. No more than two or three glasses are recommended.

Strength is a Skill

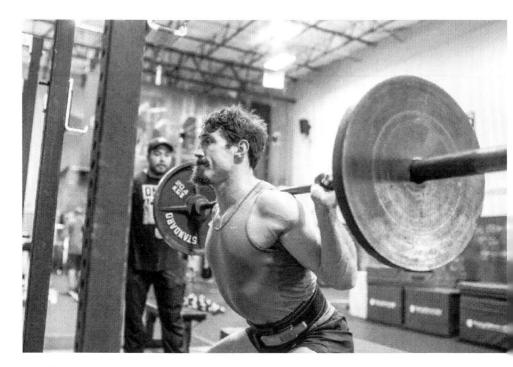

Here's a picture of Tim Kennedy. Looks like your average powerlifter Except he isn't. A former UFC fighter and member of the Marines, he is an all-round badass.

After taking off some time from fighting, he returned in late 2016 initially putting on a dominant performance. But after a round or two he got tired, gassed out, and lost the fight in shocking fashion.

In a follow up interview, he mentioned that he just didn't have it in him anymore, writing "*I felt like I was in slow motion the entire match*" This was the same guy that most Marines looked up to only days earlier. Why did this happen?

The answer is simple. Strength is a specific skill.

He spent a great deal of his time lifting weights, not fighting. Some types of strength conflict with other kinds of strength. If you want to get strong you must ask yourself this.

What do you want to get strong at? Tell a world class powerlifter to run a marathon and he won't be the best in the world at it. Tell the world's best arm wrestler to throw a hammer into the air. He will not be the best at it. You must identify what it is you want to get strong at and then adapt the contents of this book to suit that specific task.

All forms of strength fall under three basic categories. Power, speed, and endurance. For example, press-ups illustrate power and speed. Running illustrates speed and endurance.

Power is characterised by explosiveness and penetration. Powerlifting, Sprinting, and smashing the heavy bag with haymakers require power. Endomorphs, i.e. people with a pear-shaped body and wide hips and shoulders, are best suited to exerting power.

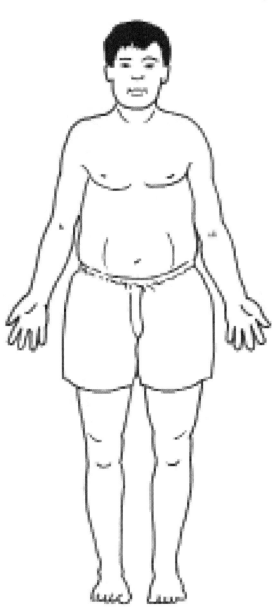

Speed relates to your reflexes and precision. Badminton and Tennis players demonstrate this. Mesomorphs, i.e. people with a wedge-shaped body, wide shoulders, narrow hips, and a minimum amount of fat, are best suited to exerting speed and agility.

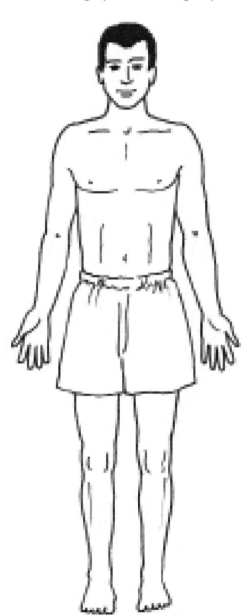

Endurance is persisting through an exercise while maintaining the same pace. Long distance races and triathlons are perfect examples. Ectomorphs, i.e. people with a streamlined and thin body, and little musculature and fat, tend to dominate endurance sports.

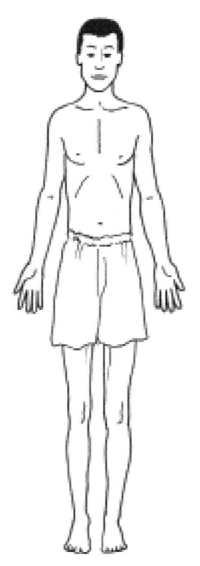

You might dispute my claim that there are body types suited to specific forms of strength. In that case, let us look at some Olympic Gold Medallists to prove my point.

rst up is a Georgian Gold Medallist Weightlifter from the 2016 lympics. His body is almost identical to the diagram of the ndomorph. Weightlifting is an explosive exercise which falls under e category of power.

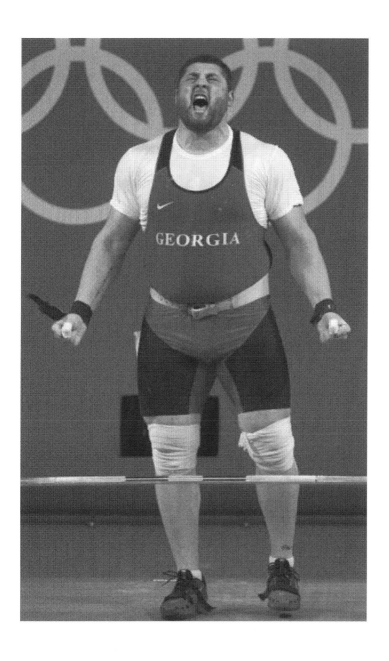

Next, comes the goalkeeper for the Danish handball team who hit gol in Rio, 2016. Handball is a sport that requires speed and skill, and littl else. Pay attention to his shoulders and hips. They replicate th Mesomorph almost exactly.

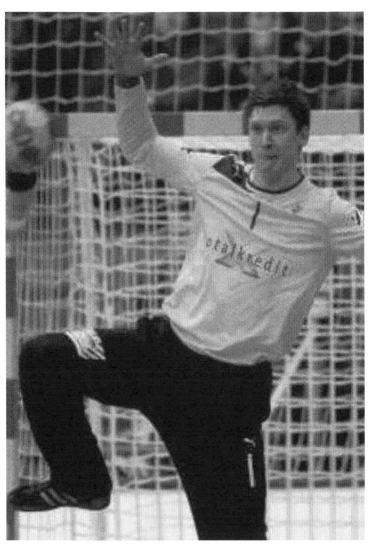

Last up is Mo Farah, the British long distance runner who set record after record, hitting Gold again in the 2016 Olympics. This time observe the roundedness of his shoulders and how streamlined his body is. There is little extra mass to carry, making his body ideal for challenging endurance activities. The perfect Ectomorph.

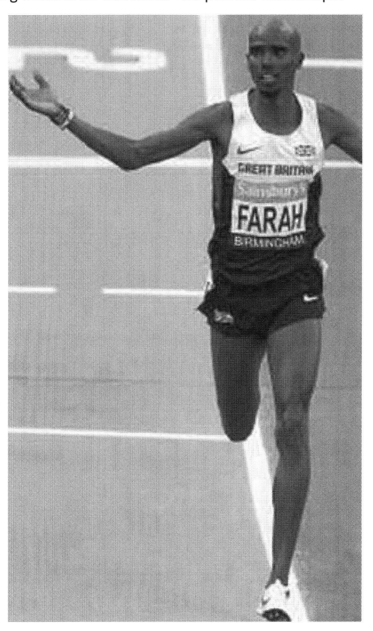

The reason I chose to look at the Gold Medallists of their respective fields is because they represent what a person can be transformed into if they specialise all their training on one specific skill.

They are the extreme. They represent the pure endomorph, mesomorph, and ectomorph.

If you identify yourself as being one kind of body type more than another, then play to your strengths and work on the matching kind of strength, e.g. if you are an endomorph use the rest of the book to improve your power as opposed to your cardio since this lies within your reach.

If you want to work on a kind of strength that is not suited to your body you will probably need to undergo an extensive transformation. Luckily for you, this book helps you improve your overall strength and fitness so you will still be able to achieve your aim but it is better for you to understand your body and work in your best interest.

There are two further classifications that can be made when talking about strength. Push and Pull. Pushing strength includes push-ups, weight lighting, and javelin throwing. Pull strength is more technical in my opinion and includes pull-ups, climbing, and cable rows.

As an example, observe this man.

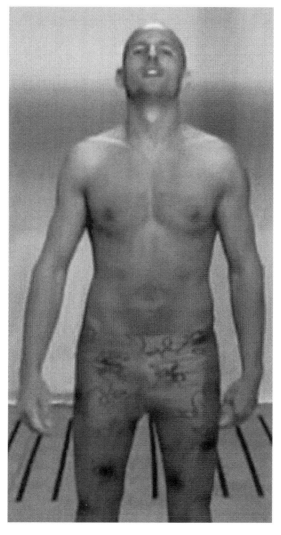

To an untrained eye, someone with great pulling strength can appear out of shape. Viewers of a YouTube video seemed confused when they saw Tazio Il Biondo, the man in the picture, perform 43 pullups in one minute. One commentator wrote:

Too bad his body doesn't look good. Looks flabby.

What the commentator had in mind was the body that you would get from pushing strength. Pushing strength works on your abdominal muscles, chest, and biceps – i.e. Arnold Schwarzenegger.

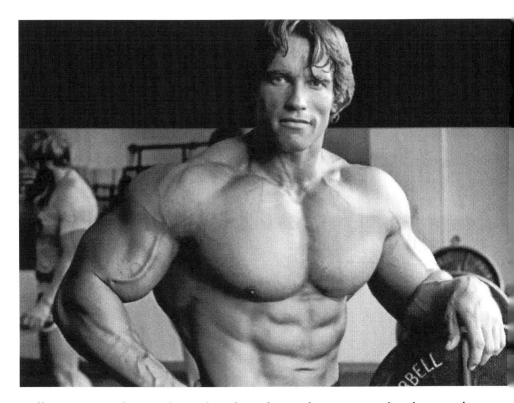

Pulling strength, on the other hand, works on your back muscles and forearms. If you were to see the same guy from the back, and compare him to a pure weight lifter, you would harbour a different opinion of his physique. In the Brazilian Jiu-Jitsu community, you will often find people with great pulling strength but not as much push strength since the martial art relies mostly on pulling your opponent's limbs. That is why their bodies are built different from that of a lifter.

Going back to the case of Tim Kennedy, commentators noticed that his physique had altered significantly since his prime fighting days. Indeed, he had moulded himself from a mesomorph into an endomorph. There were many other observations to back up the fact that he had power but lacked the strength required by a fighter, agility and endurance. I won't bore you with the details since only trained eye can infer them.

ly point stands that to get strong FAST, you need to play to your rengths. Understand your body and how you need to change or :inforce it to gain the kind of strength you seek.

my case, I was a mesomorph and wanted to become a strong appling fighter, so I did not have a conflict of interest with my body. still am a mesomorph, only a much stronger one. The route was raightforward and pain free, focusing mostly on my pull strength.

/ narrowing down on my goals, I became strong FAST, and you can o. Just note down your body type and the kind of strength you seek. e rest will play out effortlessly.

Bad Habits -- Sleeping

You want to get strong? Start by fixing all the things you're doing wrong in your life.

Sleeping affects all of us. If you sleep too little, or if you sleep too much, your strength will be affected. The optimal range of sleep for most of us is seven to eight hours. That is not all. You must time it right. You might be used to the partying life and go to sleep at four in the morning, but that is no good.

As humans, we have something called a circadian rhythm. Over thousands of years, humans have developed an internal clock in our body that adjusts itself to the Sun and the moon. Look at the diagram

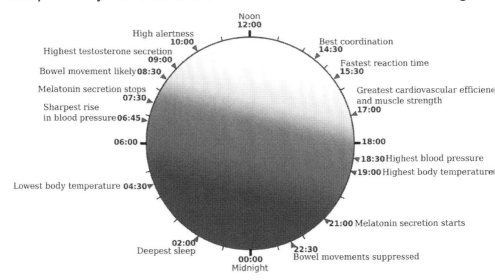

There are volumes of secrets revealed within this simple diagram that most people are unaware of. But we are looking for a specific detail.

Can you see how Melatonin secretion starts around 21:00 and stops around 07:30? Melatonin is the same chemical found within sleeping pills. It takes full effect at around 22:30 when your body suppresses bowel movements. This is the perfect time to go to sleep.

Your sharpest rise in blood pressure is around 06:45 – Just before the perfect time to wake up and be active.

Think about it. You will be forced to go to sleep eventually. By timing it right you can solve all your health and strength problems. Just do it.

A lot of younger men that I worked with noticed how their muscles became more defined when they went to bed at the right time. On top of that, timing it right meant they had an active gas tank throughout the day and would not get tired as easily. All these strength gains were thanks to sleeping at the right time, not sleeping longer. In fact, the longer you sleep the more tired you will be throughout the day!

Despite knowing all of this, I still didn't have it in me to go to sleep earlier. I preferred to doze off at four in the morning and wake up around five in the afternoon, sort of like a Vampire.

That was until I discovered that most of your time sleeping is useless. All you really need is Deep Sleep and REM Sleep. This is the portion of sleep where you typically start to dream. Before I discovered this, I would spend hours in bed waiting to fall asleep. The information overleaf on sleep cycles was life changing for me.

But be warned. The following takes some extra commitment and if you're not up to it, feel free to skip the rest of the chapter.

So how do you harness REM sleep? The answer is simple. You change your sleeping patterns. Instead of sleeping only one time in a day, you nap multiple times during the day but in shorter sessions. The reason for this is that your body will understand that it has less time to sleep and will hence try to make the most out of it. You are effectively tricking yourself into REM sleep.

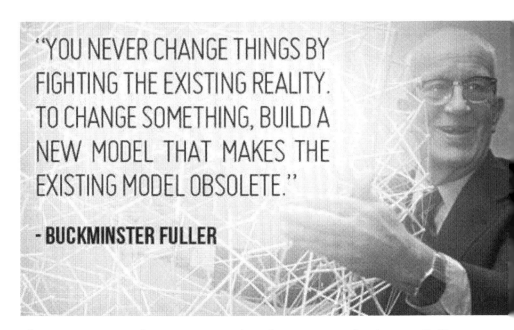

"YOU NEVER CHANGE THINGS BY FIGHTING THE EXISTING REALITY. TO CHANGE SOMETHING, BUILD A NEW MODEL THAT MAKES THE EXISTING MODEL OBSOLETE."

- BUCKMINSTER FULLER

The most astonishing case to this day was Buckminster Fuller, a true visionary. He slept for thirty minutes every six hours. After two year of following this tight regimen, doctors studied him and found him to be just fine, if not healthier than the average male.

That was only three hours of total sleep per day!

Think about it. Most people effectively spend a third of their live sleeping. Mr. Fuller only spent one eighth of his life asleep. And eve while asleep, he would really be awake since REM sleep features vivi dreams that you control. This is known as lucid dreaming.

The one thing most athletes are limited by is sleep. There is a limit t how much they can fit within a day. If Mr. Fuller had been an athlete he would have surpassed these limits beyond anything seen before.

In general, alternative sleep schedules are called Polyphasic Slee Cycles. I encourage you to look up some of them on your own, but will cover the two main ones that I recommend for improving you strength here.

The reason they improve your strength is because they act like litt doses of energy that you pick up throughout the day. Most people re on the single slot of eight hours that they get the night before. You will often see athletes complaining about their performance, saying they did not have enough sleep. If you follow a polyphasic sleep cycle, that will never be the case. You constantly charge up throughout the day and are revitalised with more and more energy whereas the people around you keep getting more and more tired.

If you've been to Spain, you know the first sleep schedule already. **Biphasic** Sleep, also known as the Siesta.

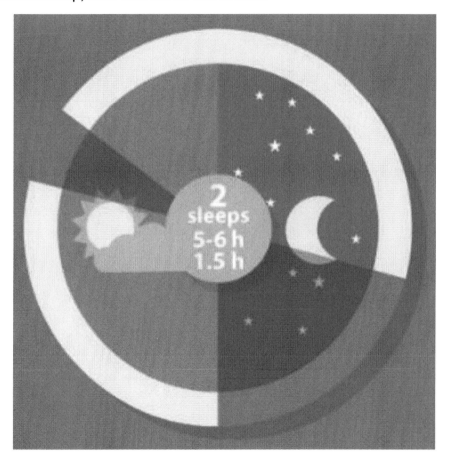

You sleep for six hours at night, and for one and a half hours after eating lunch. This can greatly improve your health in terms of cardio. What's great is that it doesn't take much time to get used to, though can be difficult to schedule.

This next schedule is much more difficult to adjust to.

The **Everyman** cycle.

After about two weeks, your body will be able to handle it and the benefits will skyrocket. But the first two weeks can be hectic. That's why I wouldn't recommend it if you have troubles with your blood pressure or have some sort of commitment such as a full-time job. Otherwise, feel free to experiment, especially during the holidays!

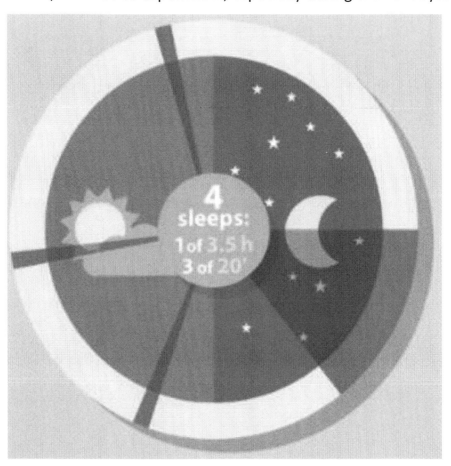

You sleep for three and a half hours at night time, and then have three further power naps – each of which takes twenty minutes. Make sure that the room you spend this time in is free from all distractions. Once you have gotten used to it, you will be fascinated by the vivid dream that the shorter naps present you with.

Personally, I tried this method for a year and became the most productive version of myself. Just think about it. You sleep for a total of four and a half hours every day. I had effectively increased my life span and had much more free time than ever before. People at my gym were puzzled as to how quickly I was improving my strength.

I stopped following it later down the road because my girlfriend insisted I sleep with her at night. Ironically, the only reason I met her was because I was awake at a time I usually would have slept through.

Scheduling your naps can be especially difficult if you do not have anywhere to rest and are on a job at noon time. Interestingly, companies such as Google and Uber understand the importance of mid-day naps and have included facilities at their respective headquarters for their employees to nap in, such as the one shown here.

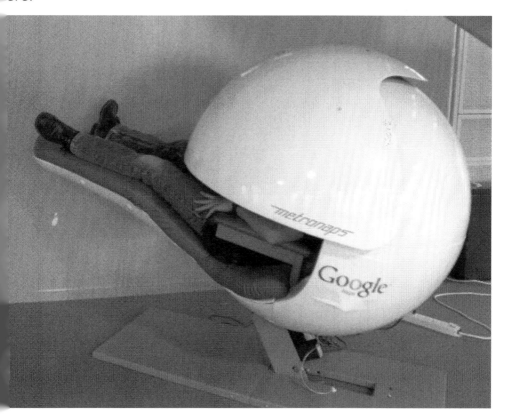

Is taking a polyphasic sleep cycle on crucial to getting strong? No. Bu it will give you an edge unlike any other. Plus, you will appreciate life more than ever before and isn't that what we all want?

Bad Habits – Drugs

Like it or not, Alcohol is a drug. Tobacco is a drug. Caffeine is a drug.

You need to understand the effects that these substances have on your body and mind, and then decide whether it's wise to moderate them.

I am not telling you to stop using them. I am asking you to not use them as often. Your first priority should be to stay sober and not surpass your limit. If you do get drunk, get drunk with friends and do it on a Friday or Saturday so that the rest of your week is not put on halt. You will have the Sunday to recover.

If you drink Coffee or a soft drink, only do so on the days you feel you will really benefit from it. And even then, moderate the number of cups you take. Make that drink count. In my experience, you cannot separate an addict from their addiction. That is why you must moderate it. This applies even to things as simple as a Pepsi bottle.

Coffee is one of the products every adult in the west loves. It is also perhaps the best mild performance enhancer out there. Check out the graph below, taken from a study by cyclingtips.com.

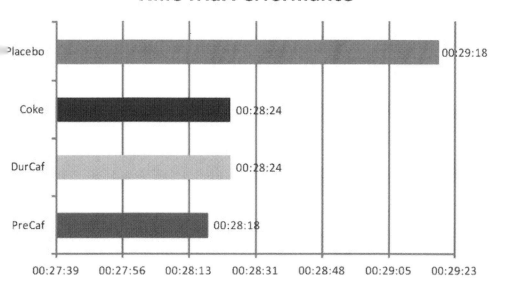

Time Trial Performance

Placebo	00:29:18
Coke	00:28:24
DurCaf	00:28:24
PreCaf	00:28:18

00:27:39   00:27:56   00:28:13   00:28:31   00:28:48   00:29:05   00:29:23

It shows the time it took for cyclists to complete a trial run while on different supplements. The placebo was just an empty pill and shows how long it would take someone to complete the race just through their physical prowess. DurCaf indicates that caffeine was consumed regularly throughout the race, whereas PreCaf indicates that caffeine was consumed one hour before the race. What the results show is that caffeine is a noticeable performance enhancer and that it has an immediate and prolonged effect on your body.

That is something most people don't realise. Drugs don't leave your body as quickly as you might think. Many athletes fail drug tests because they took cannabis a week earlier and it still had not exited their system. If you want to always be in control of your own body join me and stop using drugs altogether.

I was once doing Laundry at three in the morning when one of my flatmates at College asked me for a lighter. He had a bad dream and woke up feeling like a smoke would benefit him. I asked him whether he wanted a pack of ten Cuban cigars.

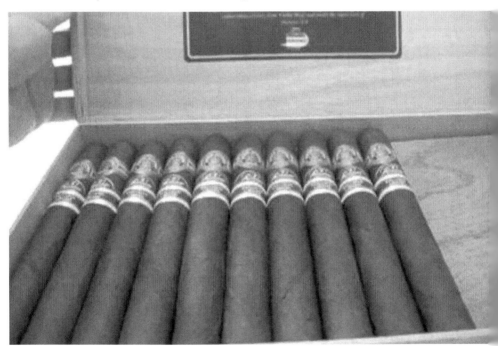

he catch was that he would have to wait until the next day to get hem. Upon receiving them, his smoking addiction halted. He used up ne cigar per week, doing so only on Fridays to mark the end of the veek. It lasted him the entire term. On his last one, he made a promise o never smoke a cigarette again.

Vith a little initiative, I had been able to help him get rid of an ddiction that he had been battling with for the past three years. His ealth steadily improved, gradually returning his full strength. If he ould do it, then so can you.

y understanding the drugs you take and cutting down on the number f times you use them, you begin to lessen the effects that these drugs ave on you. Something as simple as sugar can be addictive. Pay ttention to your surroundings and make sure you lead a balanced life.

astly, here is a drug you **do NOT** want to use to become stronger.

teroids.

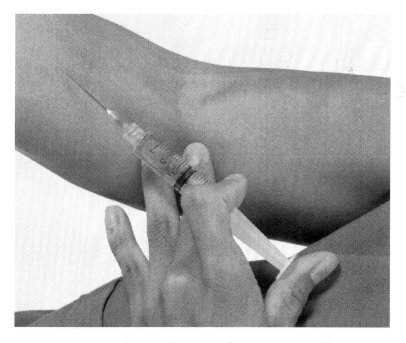

you are a guy, prolonged use of steroids will decrease your stosterone levels and shrink your testicles. I have seen too many athletes needing fertility medication because they could not get their wife pregnant due to having overused steroids in their youth. If you are still not convinced, let me point out that steroids will make you grow droopy breasts. What now?

The only time it is acceptable for a man to use steroids, is if he is in his fifties and not competing in a sport where he could seriously hurt other people. Like it or not, such a man is considered middle-aged, and can do as he sees fit. The downsides of steroids will most likely not manifest themselves within his life span, so he can take advantage of the few benefits that steroids can offer.

Here's a short aside on supplements.

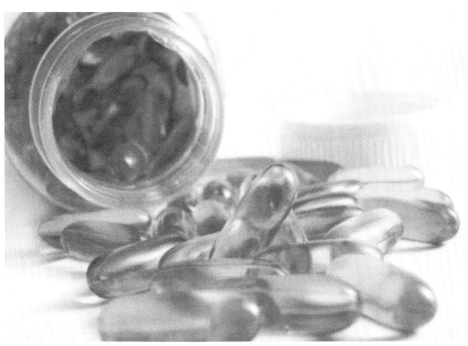

Suppose you are very pale or live somewhere with little sunlight. You might want to take Vitamin D supplements. People with other shortages in their system take a variety of supplements. Supplements are useful if you are travelling a lot and want to make sure that your body is getting the right nutrients and minerals.

Here is the problem.

he bodybuilding community might convince you to buy a surplus of
supplements. That is bad advice. Only take the ones you are sure you
re lacking in your lifestyle. For example, if you drink a lot of orange
ice already it would be useless to take a Vitamin C supplement. In
ct, it can be dangerous for your body if you do this since you might
et a surplus and disrupt your metabolism.

even Salzberg of Johns Hopkins said

> *It seems reasonable that if a little bit of something is good for*
> *you, then more should be better for you. It's not true.*
> *Supplementation with extra vitamins or micronutrients doesn't*
> *really benefit you if you don't have a deficiency.*

hink twice before buying something that a friend recommended.

Bad Habits – Masturbation

I had a friend that was addicted to masturbating. It cost him his soci
life. He seemed tired all the time and asked me how to get stronger.
told him to reduce the time he spent masturbating. Don't take it fro
me. Take it from Rickson Gracie, the greatest Brazilian Jiu-Jits
practitioner to have ever walked the face of the Planet.

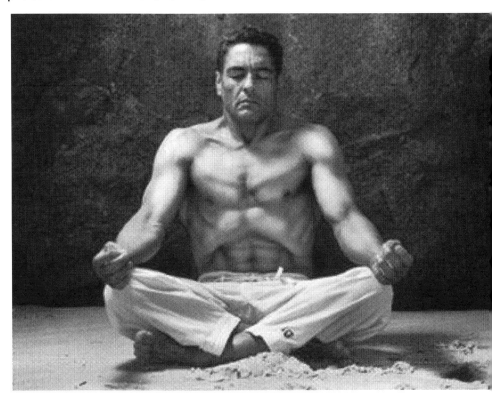

He claims that your semen contains your vital force. It is sacred ar
must not be shed without caring. Why else would athletes k
encouraged to give up masturbating months before a competition?

Aside from containing protein, semen is comprised of fructos
calcium, citric acid, magnesium, and virtually any other nutrient yc
can think of. If it does not leave your body, every single one of thos
nutrients will be reabsorbed and put to use. Just think about that.

t takes about three months for sperm to mature. If you do feel sexual needs, then satisfy them with a partner, keeping the three-month cycle in mind. Studies have shown that while sexual intercourse does lower blood pressure, among other benefits, masturbation does not.

That said, masturbation does not have any negative effects but as was the case with drugs, you must avoid an excess of it. Pornography, on the other hand, has plenty of negative side effects. Many guys get a bad understanding of what a healthy strong male looks like from watching too much Pornography. The kinds of males that partake in Pornographic content are the last thing you want to look like. To battle your addiction, join the #noFap community on Reddit if you must. The results speak for themselves.

There are thousands of stories online of boys and men reporting gains in strength from quitting masturbation once and for all.

When i was regularly fapping my i was like "fuck it man not another 10 reps, im tired".

While on noFap:"lets fucking do this! 10 reps? Bitch ill do 11! bring it on!"

This is only one example. Sadly, my friend who was addicted to masturbating never found his way out. He ended up dropping out of college. He wasted all that energy on useless things when he could have been working to improve his strength and quality of life.

That is one thing you should take away from #noFap. Do not waste your life on useless things. Make sure that every day is better than the last one. The first step to achieving this is to quit your bad habits.

Now that that is over, it is time to reveal the secrets of strength to you.

Secrets of Strength – Breathing

I am about to reveal to you the first secret. When I first discovered this, it changed everything. Here is the guy who taught it to me.

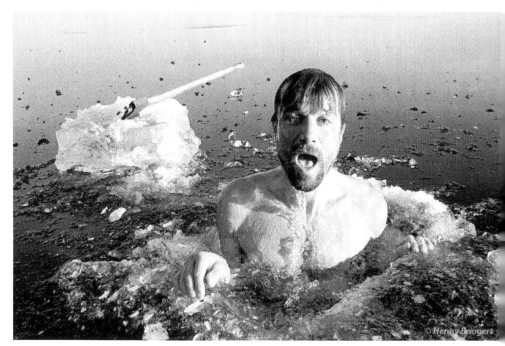

His name is Wim Hof, though most people know him as The Ice Man. He has run marathons on the arctic circle. In his underwear. Most people assume he works out. He doesn't. The secret to his strength is the Wim Hof breathing method.

Most will learn his method to try and achieve enlightenment, or some other fancy goal. The problem is, they get carried away by his teaching methods. I will tell you exactly how to use it to get strong FAST.

But first, here is a question. Why do you get tired?

Fitness trainers will tell you it is because you do not exercise often enough. But the truth lies inside your blood. You are running short of oxygen. You become tired because your brain tries to make sure that your oxygen levels don't run too low and cause you to pass out.

Now for the big takeaway. What would happen if you somehow managed to supercharge your blood with oxygen? You would never run low on fuel, and therefore never get tired! That is what the Wim Hof method tries to do. Use your breath to increase your strength.

will first be getting you to do the breathing method. By the end of it ou may feel light headed and experience a tingling or electrical ensation. Then I will tell you how it can make you strong FAST.

it down comfortably and breathe easily without any pressure. The ey here is to reach a baseline, and find a natural pose. You might want o lie down, or sit on the side of your bed. I prefer the side of my bed. our body should feel relaxed with your back kept straight.

egin by breathing from your abdominal area, working to your lungs. you are like most people, you will breathe from your chest. That is o good. You want to first inflate your stomach like a balloon.

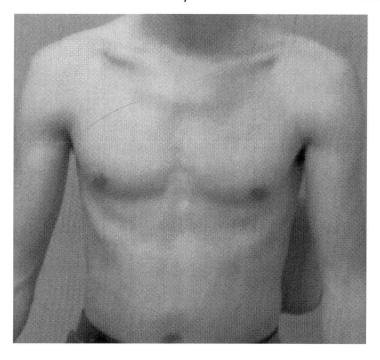

If you find it difficult, watch a few videos on diaphragmatic breathing
Once your stomach has been inflated, fill up your lungs with air unti
they are completely full, feeling your upper sides expand.

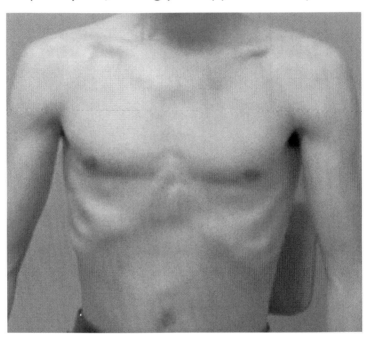

The aim is to breathe in as deeply as possible without having to forc
it. You're your sternum pushing against your chest. To help, keep
straight back and consider opening your mouth wide as you breathe
Your body is like a balloon and you need to fill it up. Once full, hold
for a moment.

Breathe out easily, but don't overdo it. You want to have air lef
Your body should return back to its baseline.

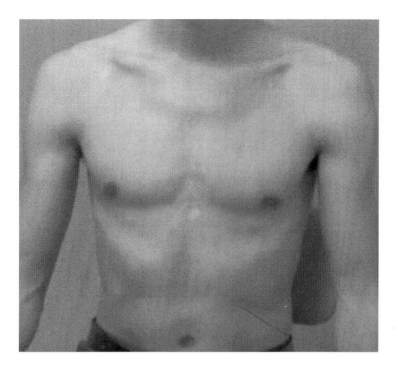

he whole point of this exercise is to have more oxygen stay in your
loodstream than before. Deep inhalations leave some oxygen inside
our body. By breathing out too deeply, this is exhaled without having
een exchanged to carbon dioxide. That is why you do not exhale too
uch, just enough to return to the baseline you had in the first step.
principle, this can be likened to a controlled hyperventilation.

epeat this until you feel saturated with oxygen, ideally thirty times.
veryone is different. Do no push past your limits, but aim for thirty.

reathe in for one last time, exhale completely and then hold it.
mediately after the thirty, breathe in deeply one last time. Then
xhale completely and hold this breath. Make sure to tuck your chin
not let any air out by accident. Once you feel the gasp reflex at the
p of your chest, you can breathe out. But aim to hold it for a while.

eathe fully for recovery. Hold this last breath for fifteen seconds.
aving gasped for air after holding your breath, you now breathe in
lly one last time and hold it for around fifteen seconds. Feel your

chest expand. Once your body tells you to let go of the breath, let go. You will know to let go when you feel your heart pounding heavily.

You have now completed one round. Aim to do a round per day to get used to the breathing pattern so that you can use it later on.

Although I told you to hold your breath for fifteen seconds, you should try to hold it for longer every day. This breath retention is important. The longer you can hold it **comfortably**, the more oxygen your body must be able to hold.

When you hold your breath, there is a moment when your blood vessels constrict and become thin. Pressure accumulates.

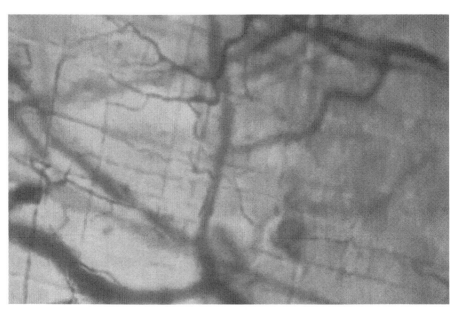

The moment you breathe out, this blood rushes through and circulates. Your blood vessels dilate. If this blood has already been oxygenated with the breathing method beforehand, you will have quickly circulated oxygen to your whole body!

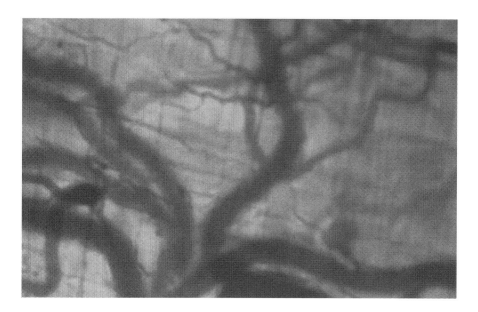

Here is the question you have been waiting for. How can you use all of this to gain superhuman strength? Let's take the example of push-ups. If you can do ten push-ups while holding your breath, then how many can you do while breathing? Way more.

Complete four cycles of the breathing method. On the fourth cycle, hold your breath and perform as many push-ups as you can. Do this every two to three days at most. You can do this as little as once a week and still see incredible results.

When holding your breath, you should pay attention to how the blood circulates in your body. This is something you must feel for yourself.

Once you are rested from the push ups, perhaps a day or two later, you might be interested to see how strong you have gotten. Perform four cycles of the breathing method and then do as many push-ups as you can while breathing. Note how much easier it has gotten since you were able to do them while holding your breath.

This exercise can be adapted to any form of strength training. Later, you can take the example of running – but not to begin with since the risk of getting light headed while running and then falling and hurting yourself is not worth it.

Here is my story with this method. There was an incredibly hot girl fancied during High school. My plan was to win the four-kilometr race on Sports Day, then ask her out on a high note. The only problem was I had never run more than a hundred metres before.

And the other guys were much more athletic than I would ever be.

The day before the race, I went to the track when no one was ther and started to run. I gassed out after thirty paces. That was when thought to pay more attention to my breath. Without knowing it, I di the Wim Hof method while running. I breathed in deeply every two paces then exhaled a bit for the other two paces.

While running, my mind felt separate from my body and I had sensation of coldness around my chest. While my legs did hurt, I n longer felt tired. At least not physically. However, my brain wa confused and felt like it should be tired. I quickly focused my mind c the task and promised myself that I would not quit. This was the ke step. You must remember this. Commit to the task. Another lap.

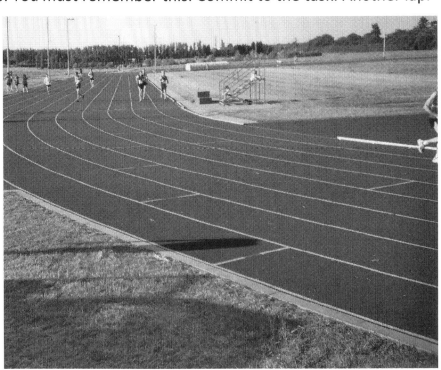

lowly, my legs began to relax as well. No tension. I went on to achieve rst place in the race, but still did not understand how I did it. I was oo caught up in studying my breathing and forgot to ask the girl out. few weeks later I discovered Wim Hof. My life was never the same.

have taught this method to many friends, some of whom were nitially asthmatic. The only time they could not run further was ecause they were not committed to the task. I asked one of my iends why he stopped running and he told me that he didn't feel red but he felt like he wanted to stop.

his is known as mental exhaustion. Your brain thinks you should be red, but your body isn't thanks to the Wim Hof method. That is why ou stop even though you could go on for many more miles. If you find ourself experiencing this, read the next chapter which will teach you ow to discipline your mind and overcome mental challenges.

Secrets of Strength – Embrace the Cold

Cold temperature is an uncomfortable and often unbearable experience for most of us. You attribute the cold to sickness and toughness. Hard going countries such as Russia and Norway are known for their cold temperatures as well as the tough and well-built men they produce. It's true. Exposing yourself to cold temperatures strengthens your mind and body in a unique way.

Cold weather will make you sick.

That statement is a lie! What really happens is your body tends to produces more *genes* which trigger inflammation during the winter. This causes swelling and a general feeling of unease, which is a defence mechanism to protect you from most germs. However, it is also a relatively useless reaction.

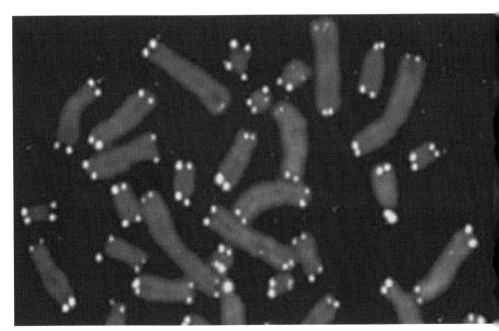

In African countries where temperatures are warm all year, people bodies produce these same genes during the rainy season when the air is damp and malaria as well as other infections are more likely to spread. Do you want your body to get weak during the winter? No nat is why you must rewire your body and intentionally expose ourself to the cold. Doing so strengthens your immune system.

also strengthens your mind. If you have never done this before, it is credibly difficult to get your mind to cope. The first time I tried to ep into a cold shower, I stood there for half an hour staring at the unning water. When I finally got in, my core tensed up and my jaw arted to shake.

felt like I had to keep my brain from jumping out of my skull.

/hen I was done, I went out for a run. This time my mind no longer It tired. I looked out into the distance and told myself I would keep oing. My head was still tense from the cold shower. It had ndamentally changed me.

nere is also another secret most athletes know about nowadays but on't use properly. Active recovery. Here is a question. If I locked you a gym, gave you food, and told you to become as strong as Mike /son, or I won't let you back out to your normal life, would you train I the time? Yes. Since you have nothing better to do and want to sume your life, you would probably try to train without a break. But e truth is that doing so is counterproductive!

'hen you work out too often, your body stops becoming stronger and st stays as it is.

ne reason for this is that lactic acid and other toxins accumulate ound your muscles and slow down their growth. Someone who orks out seven times a day will be just as good as someone that orks out only once a day. He might even get worse in the long run as e lactic acid continues to build up.

ne only way to make sure that all your training is really benefiting you by exposing your body to cold ice or water.

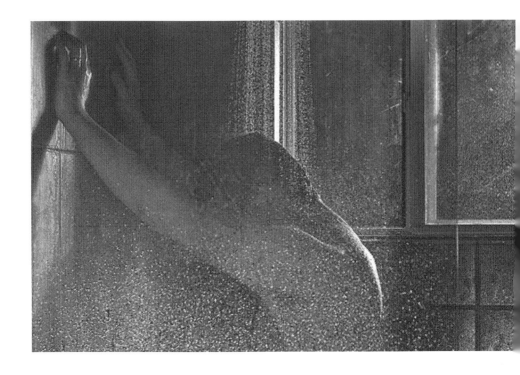

The coldness will constrict your blood vessels and cleanse your body of lactic acid. Then when you go back to room temperature, your blood transports oxygen to these areas so they continue to grow and strengthen the next time you train.

There are two ways to expose yourself to the cold. Either a Cold shower, or a hardcore ice bath. I prefer the ice bath but it takes time and money to prepare. When you start out, a cold shower will do. It is best to follow my method written here if you want all the benefits described.

Here are some instructions on how to set up the ice bath for the future. Buy two or three bags of ice from a convenience store.

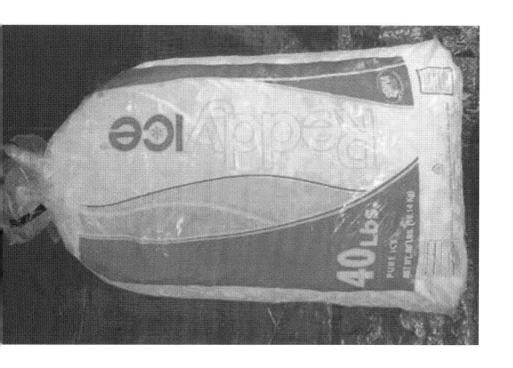

ll your bath tub up halfway with cold water. Then fill it up with the
e and give the water a minute or two to drop in temperature. Move
e ice around to make sure that it is evenly distributed. If you want
 enter the ice bath, make sure to wear shorts so that your crotch
ea remains healthy. You do not want to dramatically change the
mperature of your penis. It is too sensitive.

 enter the ice bath, first enter your legs to get used to it. While
ing the Wim Hof method, visualise the oxygen circulating through
ur legs. Sit down and as you do first enter your right side and then
ur left side. Settle into the bath but make sure that your head is
icking out.

ur head must stick out. And you must stay alert throughout the Ice
th.

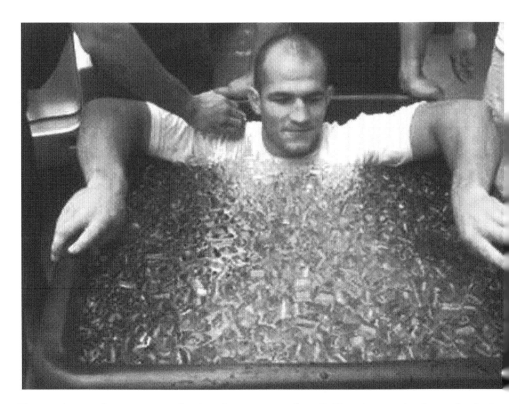

There have been people in the past who fell asleep during their Ice Bath while submerged in the water up to their mouth and nearly drowned. Remember to only stay within the Ice Bath for ten to twenty minutes. Do not go past twenty minutes so as to avoid frostbites and other unpleasant side effects.

Your body might be shaking. Your goal is to feel yourself and the flow of blood within you. Try to concentrate on the warmth within you to keep your body temperature constant. After a few tries, you might want to start to hold your breath while doing this. Feel your heart pounding vigorously against the ice water. It's an amazing experience.

I will now describe how to get into the **Cold Shower**.

Before you start the cold treatment, do the Wim Hof method. Fill your blood with extra oxygen, but make sure that you are fully awake.

When you feel slightly light headed, focus on the tension in your forehead and enter the shower headfirst. Then turn around and

xpose your back to the cold water. You will be surprised by how little
ou register the temperature on your head and back.

inally, turn around to expose your sides to the water – indicated by
ie blue marks on the picture.

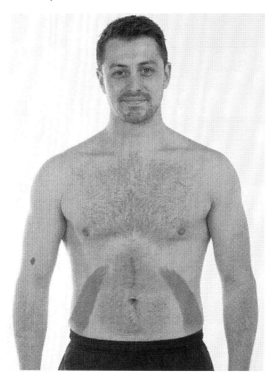

iis will require the most courage from you. You might feel your
uscles spasm if you are sensitive. Keep breathing as you do. Make
re that your entire body has been exposed to the water.

you are fighting masturbation addiction, run cold water on your
nitals every night.

summarise, you can take a cold treatment after training to recover,
fore training to prepare your mind for perseverance, or to work on
ur breath holding abilities.

ou need extra motivation to commit to it every day, know that Wim
f has done it in the Arctic – after smashing the ground with an axe.

If he can do it, then so can you.

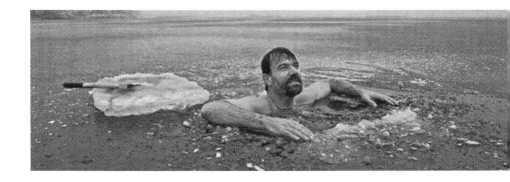

ecrets of Strength – Tabata Protocol

Vhat if I told you that there is a way to do four minutes of work and xperience the same gains as someone putting in hours at the gym.

Vell, there is.

umi Tabata is your typical crazy scientist. He solved our problem. ow to get strong FAST. And a lot of people are doing it wrong.

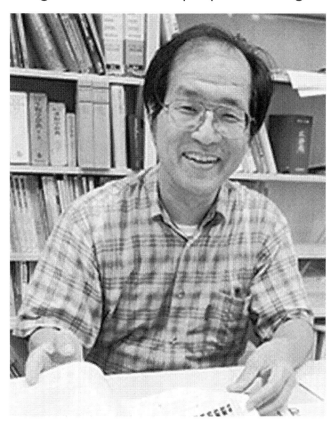

im Hof will improve your endurance to superhuman levels. But it will ot do much as far as your raw explosive strength and muscle mass e concerned. That is where Tabata comes in handy.

ink back to earlier in the book where I wrote that Olympic athletes e the best at what they do. In fact, they are so good that it is often possible for them to continue improving at a noticeable rate – since they have already achieved peak physical condition. This is wha everyone thought until Tabata hit the scene.

Olympic speed skating is a gruelling sport where athletes spend hour in the gym every single day trying to improve their cardiovascula strength.

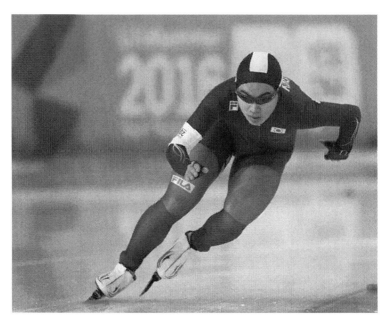

Yet all those hours were shown to be ineffective.

After spending only four minutes with a group of athletes, Tabat managed to significantly improve their VO2 Max. The VO2 Max is measure of how well your body can absorb oxygen while undergoir a specific exercise. Think about it. If your body consumes more oxyge during an exercise, which builds on certain muscles, then thos muscles will continue to grow.

When I first heard about this, I quickly tried to focus my Taba workout only on my arms. I wanted arms as big as Arno Schwarzenegger. That was a mistake. I soon realised how difficult th four minute Tabata workout can be. It is much better to go for a fu body workout and improve your full body strength. Let me give yc the full story. At the time, I was trying to beat my Sports Teacher whe hrowing a javelin. When I threw my javelin, it would travel half as far s when my teacher threw it. His arms were twice the size of mine and early, he had much more practice than I did.

n an attempt beat him, I began to follow a Tabata styled workout hich focused on my arms, hips, and legs. After only two weeks, I saw najor improvements in my strength. I swung the javelin with my arm, while pushing back on the ground with my legs and twisting my hips rith great power. My javelin landed half a foot in front of that of my eacher, who was left gobsmacked. Ever since, I have been trying to increase awareness for the Tabata Protocol. It did not take me years o make such a great improvement. Only four minutes of hard work, aree to five days a week.

efore you begin, you must think of a set of simple exercises, referably **four**. If overall strength is what you seek, make sure that ne simple exercises cover your full body, e.g. bicep curls for your ms, sit-ups for your abdominal muscles, pull-ups for your back, and quats for your legs.

ake sure they are simple exercises. You should be able to pull off at east a dozen in a time of twenty seconds, if you work hard enough. ny exercise incorporating your own bodyweight, free weights, or a weighted vest work just fine.

ou will also need a ten-minute warm up plan before starting. **This is ucial**. Without it, the Tabata Protocol fails. Warming up should get our muscles and joints loose and allow for blood to flow to your uscles. It is best to make the warm up specific to your strength aining. For example, I warm up specifically to my Brazilian Jiu-Jitsu aining by incorporating rolling around and leg stretches. However, if u ironically are too lazy to design a warmup, there is a general warm plan coming up.

t's jump the gun!

For each exercise, you will:

1. Do the exercise for 20 seconds at the highest possible intensity
2. Rest for 10 seconds
3. Repeat these two steps eight times

Overall, you're only spending four minutes on the exercise. For the first step, you **must** take it literally. Perform the exercise as explosively and as fast as is physically possible. Do not slowdown at any time during these twenty seconds.

You must explode!

When I was doing sit-ups as part of my Tabata training, my abdominal muscles hurt like hell. I was going all out and sweating gallons while doing so. You must be completely committed to the task. Sure, hurts. But it is only twenty seconds at a time.

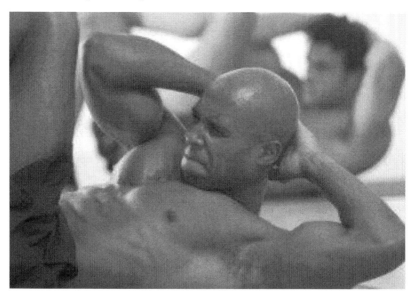

The original Tabata regimen only featured intense cycling as i exercise. However, moderate weightlifting, sprinting, and dynamic bodyweight exercises – such as pull-ups, sit-ups, and burpees – are acceptable as well as many more. Note that stationary exercises, such as holding the plank, will not work.

fter a while, I got sick of the pain the Tabata method put me through. was then that I had an idea which took the Tabata Protocol to new vels. My crazy thought was to **perform the Wim Hof method during e ten second rest periods**. To no surprise, it worked even better!

oing this will help you get strong FAST and EASY.

***

General Warm Up Plan (10 minutes)

ere's a sample warm up plan designed to be as effective, simple, and on-specific as possible while taking up approximately ten minutes of our time. It warms up most of the body, but you should change it to e more specific to the kinds of activities you plan to do within the ibata Protocol.

egin by stretching your **ankles** as shown. Sit back and roll on the balls your feet, shifting your bodyweight forwards and backwards until u feel loose in your joints. Focus on your ankles, as well as your toes.

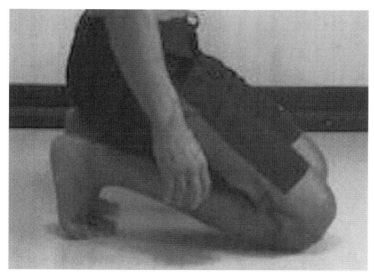

ext, sit on your shins. This stretch targets your ankles and your ees. Hold this stretch for a minute or longer. If you are not asonably flexible, this will hurt a lot. To increase the stretch, lean or backwards.

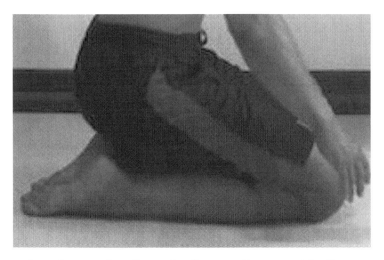

Place your hands on the floor in front of you with fingers pointing towards your knees and palms facing up. Pulse the pressure that you apply to the joint. Make sure it is not stiff and does not click by the end.

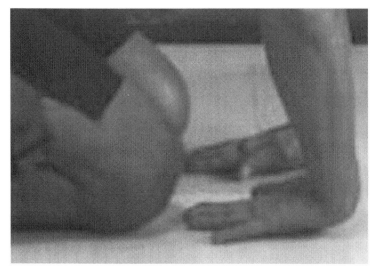

Reverse your hands so that your palms are facing the ground this time around. Again, pulse the pressure applied to the joint. Make sure that your thumbs are on the outside, not the inside. By the end of the minute your **wrists** should feel loose.

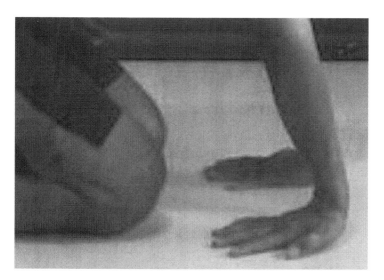

ow assume the bridge position. This will moderately stretch your ps and work to engage your **core**. Hold it for three seconds and rest r a second. Then repeat fifteen times.

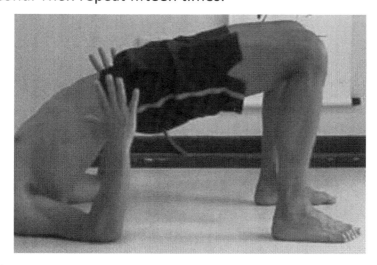

u might want to twist your **hips** left and right to get rid of any clicks at could hinder performance during the Tabata protocol. Hold for irty seconds and when you feel uncomfortable, drop to either side your body before resuming.

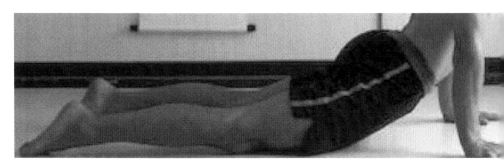

Stretch your **lower back**. To not get hurt during this, ease into the stretch and make sure that your hips and spine are aligned well. To make it more difficult, stand on your toes.

Next, relieve tension from your **neck** by holding each of the following stretches for half a minute.

First tuck your chin towards your chest to stretch the back of the neck.

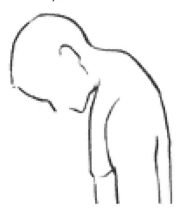

Then, look up towards the ceiling, or even back further if you can.

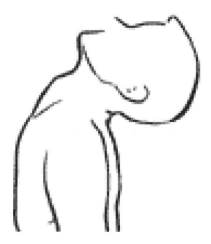

ove your left ear towards your left shoulder, but don't overdo it.

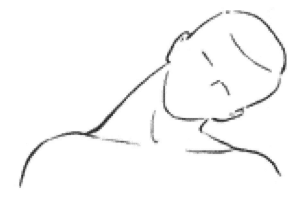

nally, move your right ear towards your right shoulder.

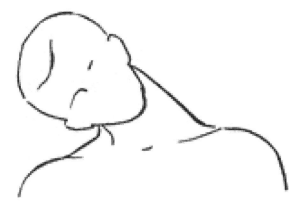

uch your chin to your left shoulder, supporting your head with your
nd if you need to.

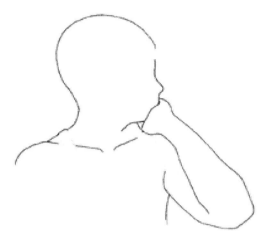

Finally, touch your chin to your right shoulder.

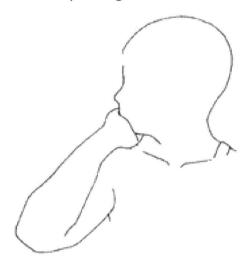

For your final stretch, roll your **shoulders** in full circles forwards ar
backwards, raising your shoulders as high as your ears. Do this fiftee
times both going forwards and backwards.

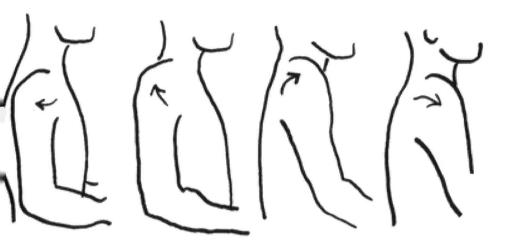

nce fully stretched, start **running** on the spot for two to three full
inutes. First at low intensity, then gradually raising your pace and
nees higher and higher. If your thighs feel painful, simply lower your
nees and pace. Swing your arms along with your legs.

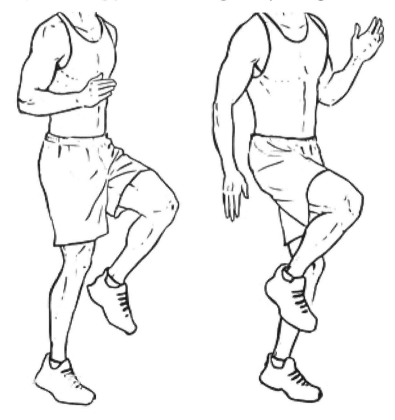

Jump up and down a full twenty times. Instead of bending your knee to jump, flick your feet up and down, to propel yourself upwards on the balls of your feet. This will contract your legs and shock your **shin bones** upon landing, thus strengthening them. Your heart rate should be raised significantly by the end of this. If it isn't, jump up and down a further twenty times.

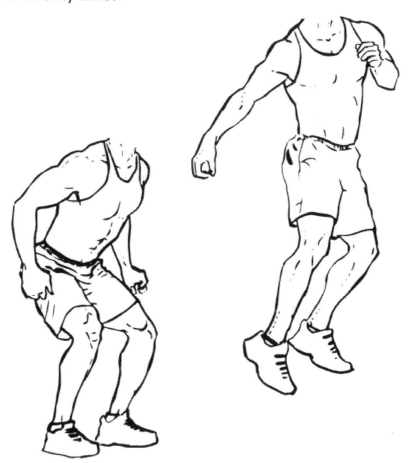

Lower the height at which you jump, but this time land in a full squat. Make sure to land as deeply as possible, preferably with your **buttocks** touching your ankles if you can. Exhale deeply when landing in the squat. Repeat a full twenty times, keeping good form.

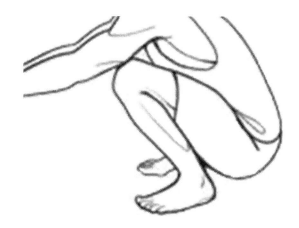

our legs may feel dead after all this jumping, so perform ten forward
g swings to get the blood rushing again and to open your hips. Let
our legs undergo a full 180-degree range of motion. You might want
• hold on to something if you do not have a good sense of balance.
aise your legs slower and slower as you progress. The slower you do,
•e more control of your leg muscles you show.

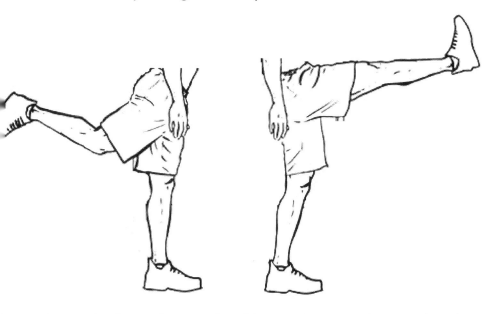

ow swing each of your legs to the side ten times, again ensuring that
•ey undergo a full 180-degree rotation if you can. On your tenth one,
• to raise your leg as slowly as possible while raising it as high as you
•n. This will put your leg muscles to the test.

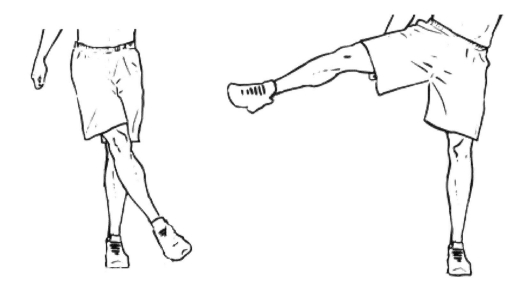

Stand naturally, then fall into a full lunge while twisting your body to either side. Repeat twenty times. This engages your **hips** and **core**. Avoid doing these fast, focusing more on the penetration of the stretch as well as the twist of the hips.

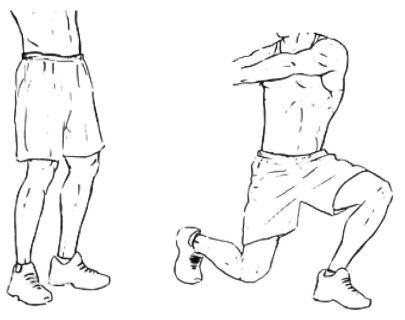

To finish the warmup and get ready to become a real-life Superman, perform twenty repetitions of the Superman pose. Lie down, and the ill your legs and arms off the floor by flexing your **core**. Hold for three five seconds and rest for a second. Repeat twenty times.

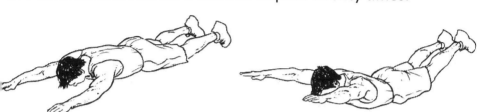

is concludes the general warmup plan. Unlike most warmup plans does not contain sit-ups or press-ups, since these will most likely be rt of your Tabata exercise and would reduce your ability to perform em when needed.

***

Sample Tabata Workout Plan

ere, I will give you the Tabata workout that I first practiced when I ed to improve my Javelin throwing abilities. It should give you an ea of how to develop your own Tabata workout, but should not be pied blindly if it does not work on the parts of the body that you int to strengthen. Also note that it uses gym equipment that you will obably not have access to at home, although the Tabata workout es not need to be done with gym equipment.

Warmup – 10 minutes.

Exercise 1

Cycling Machine – 20 seconds

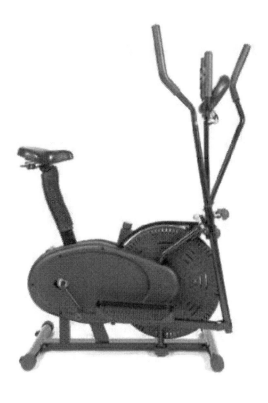

Rest and Breathe – 10 seconds

Repeat two previous steps eight times (x8)

Alternative: Jump rope

xercise 2

able Core Rotation – 20 seconds

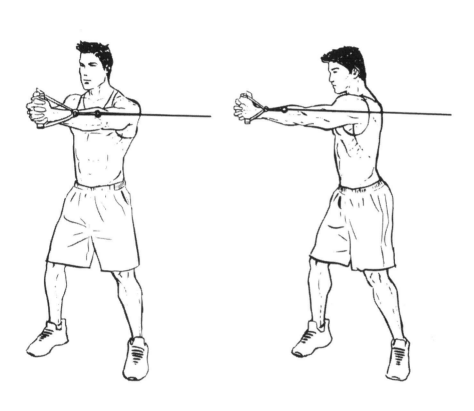

est and Breathe – 10 seconds

epeat two previous steps eight times (x8)

ternative: Throw a medicine ball at the wall.

Exercise 3

Jumping Lunges – 20 seconds

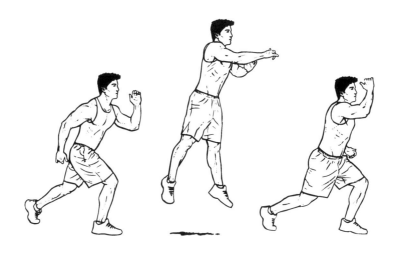

Rest and Breathe – 10 seconds

Repeat two previous steps eight times (x8)

The key to this exercise is to focus on exploding upwards and ⌐
landing safely. Make sure to ease into a full lunge before explodi█
upwards again at full power. This exercise will wonders for your le▁
and there is no other substitute for this kind of jump training.

xercise 4

ettlebell Swings – 20 seconds

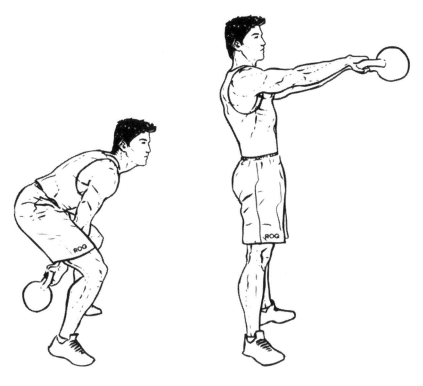

est and Breathe – 10 seconds

epeat two previous steps eight times (x8)

Cool down – 2 minutes

What do you do in the cooldown? Gently shake your arms and legs t make sure they are loose. This is the best time to stretch since you muscles have been loosened up. Take an ice bath or cold showe straight afterwards if you don't want sore muscles.

Let me say this again. You must go all out when doing these exercise All or nothing.

ecrets of Strength – Visualisation

ave you ever heard people say that if you visualise your desire it will
me true? At first, I did not buy into it.

ıt then, I saw Conor McGregor (the former UFC featherweight and
htweight champion) accidentally mention it in an interview. After
illing the details, he looked like he had revealed one of his biggest
crets and somewhat regretted doing so. Sure enough, all the things
claimed to have visualised came true within the following year.

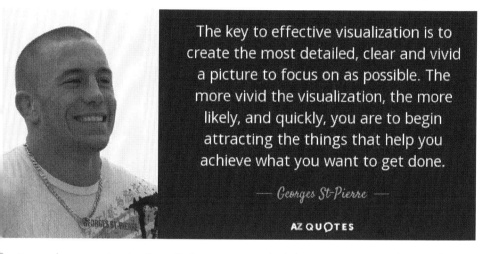

The key to effective visualization is to
create the most detailed, clear and vivid
a picture to focus on as possible. The
more vivid the visualization, the more
likely, and quickly, you are to begin
attracting the things that help you
achieve what you want to get done.

— Georges St-Pierre —

AZ QUOTES

hat made me start visualising my goals however was when I found
t GSP (former UFC Welterweight and Middleweight Champion) had
ıted the same much earlier.

fore I dive in deep into this subject, I want to give you a simple task.

ɔm now on, start all your exercises by visualising the outcome. For
ample, let's say you are going to do push-ups. Calmly sit with your
es closed and visualise yourself performing the push-ups first. See
ur body and feel your biceps contracting and relaxing as your breath
culates blood through your body and you work to complete the
ercise. Visualise yourself successfully completing the exercise
thout getting tired and doing so smoothly and with ease.

You will be surprised at the sense of familiarity you will experience when you later do the actual exercise, having visualised it beforehand

Scientists have broken this down into a four-step process. Let us take the example of a simple pull-up.

1. Visualise the pull-up you are going to do and the goal you want to achieve and see yourself achieving it. The more vivid this is the better the results.
2. Just before you are about to perform the pull-up, visualise yourself successfully performing the pull-up. This is right before you will perform the pull-up, as you reach for the bar.
3. Repeat the same visualisation while performing the pull-up. This can be kind of difficult, but make sure to not close your eyes as you want to observe yourself performing the movement.
4. Finally, visualise the pull-up you just performed – the actual event. Use this actual event as a guideline to strengthen future visualisations. If you identified a problem in your form, visualise another pull-up in which you have corrected this then try again

In general, you visualise the pull-up before and during the exercise then replay the actual exercise in your mind and use it to strengthen the visualisation or autocorrect it in your mind if it did not go per plan

This was the common method researched by Scientists. However there are many secrets they did not research as thoroughly.

Here is a method to achieving an adrenaline rush that will give you boosts of strengths by playing on past failures. Inevitably, when performing a tough exercise – such as dead-lifting a heavy weight you will fail in the beginning. Suppose you want to perform the same exercise again. First, visualise yourself failing and how it makes you feel. Visualise a person you care about, or an attractive partner scoffing at you. Absorb the feeling of anger, motivation, and adrenaline that results from this, and perform the exercise.

owever, this method of achieving the adrenaline rush should only be ed immediately prior to performing the exercise, since the effect is t prolonged. Also, do not use it too frequently, only when you are tempting to surpass new limits.

e most powerful form of visualisation is within the Lucid dream. This ppens when you are aware that you are dreaming and can affect e dream world directly. I can easily get into this state. There are ys for you to achieve this. I encourage you to look some up online. owever, you can manifest this ability naturally by following the cond sleep schedule mentioned in an earlier Chapter.

ientists studied Lucid dreamers and discovered that performing ks in the dream world activate the same neural pathways that uld be activated if you were to perform the task in the real world.

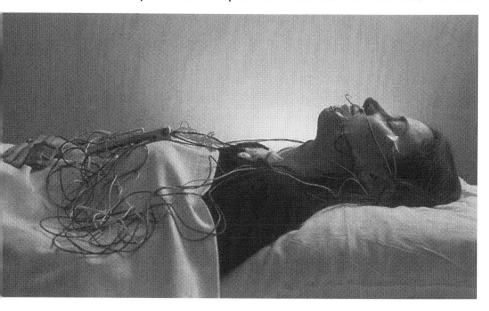

woman having an orgasm in the dream world will show the same ysiological changes in the real world. The following is not eudoscience. Experiments were done on avid lucid dreamers.

nan playing basketball in the dream world will improve his real-rld basketball skills. While working out in your dream will not make u stronger, it will improve your fine motor skills. Thus, if you want to work on your weightlifting technique, football striking technique or your wrestling technique, doing it within your lucid dream can help tremendously. The reason for this is the dream state is nearly indistinguishable from real life experience.

Suppose you are very bad at visualising. Then you can try something like to call physical assumption. As a man seeking improved strength you want to boost your testosterone levels. This is the natural hormone that makes men stronger than women.

Well guess what, there is a way to increase it up to 20% for significant periods of time by virtually standing still. That's a twenty-percent testosterone boost!

To reap this superpower, you must assume a "superman power pose" while *feeling* an aura of power. Settle in to the feel of the pose. Assume the awesomeness that comes along with it. Here is Clark Kent holding the Superman Power Pose.

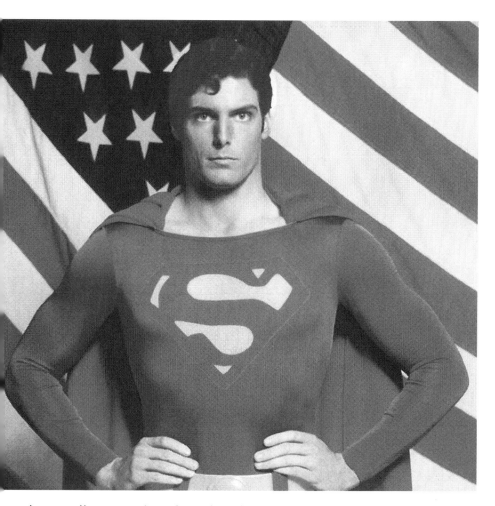

ısed to walk around with a slouched pose and this worked against
e in social situations where I would be shy and uncomfortably,
ɒically with my back to the wall. Whenever I needed to do
mething nerve-wracking that called upon my strength, I would run
a private area and stand in The Awesome Superman Pose for thirty
conds with my head held high and my chest struck out – breathing
the awesome air. Immediately, I would feel much more confident
d run back to society ready to deliver an ass-kicking. It really works!

ere were follow-up studies done, noticeably by Zurich University, in
attempt to discredit such a power pose. What they did not account
r was the feeling. Simply holding the pose is half the work. Feel the

awesomeness and superiority that comes along with it, and enjoy free boost of 20% in testosterone!

ecrets of Strength – The Russian Secret

oviet Russia had its downs but ultimately gave birth to the greatest
eightlifters of their time, some of whom still hold records. The next
ecret to be revealed within this book makes traditional weightlifting
bsolete. But be warned. If you cannot commit to a simple plan, this
not for you. If you can, you will experience immense strength gains.

ere is Pavel Tsatsouline.

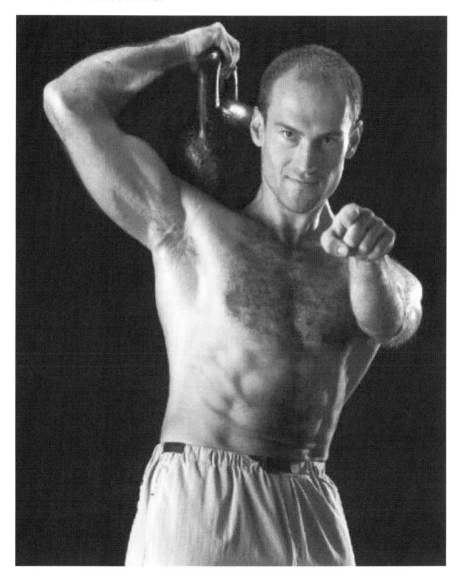

Here he is shown holding a **Kettlebell**. The ultimate conditioning tool for FAST strength gains. I will never ask you to join a gym or buy a set of weights. What I will have you consider is buying a Kettlebell. In his book, Pavel claimed,

You can replace an entire gym with a couple of kettlebells.

If you are an average male, get yourself a **sixteen** or **twenty-four kilogram** kettlebell depending on whether you can lift it at all. In the future, you might want a thirty-two kilogram one.

For females, eight, twelve or sixteen-kilogram kettlebells might be worth trying out since feminine physiques vary widely and it is difficult to give consistent advice. The upper echelons will need twenty or twenty-four kilogram kettlebells.

When training with kettlebells, there are a few key pieces of advice that you need to remember.

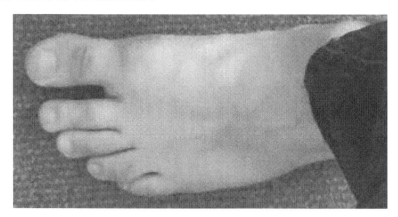

First off, <u>always</u> train **barefoot**. If you can't, then at the very least strive to wear flat and thin soled shoes, or socks. There must be room for your toes to spread and adjust your balance. Having a good grip the floor is very important.

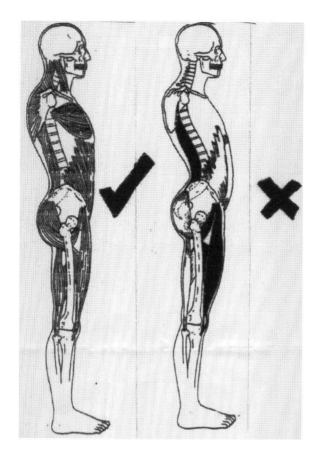

ce this is a form of lifting weights, it is important to **have a strong
ck**. Avoid flexing your spine, or performing forward and backward
nding stretches. Try to keep a straight back and decent posture. The
ssure of the Kettlebell on your misaligned spine is a problem.

vays train in a **large space** where you can swing your arms and legs
ely without bumping into objects or other people. Trust me, you
I get hurt if you exercise in a small space. I once lost my balance
ring an exercise and had a whole bookshelf fall on me

ou get incredibly tired and you start to breathe heavily, **don't stop
oving** altogether. Keep moving around exercising lightly until your
art rate slows down to an acceptable level to avoid problems with
Jr heart and blood pressure due to a sudden drop in motion.

ally, **focus on the quality** of your movements, **not the quantity**. I
going to reveal to you a few simple movements that you need to

perform daily. If you do the basic movement incorrectly, that will ge
you nowhere. If you do the basic movement, but slower than
stronger person, or with less repetitions then at least you know yo
will be getting stronger. Do everything correctly.

Now for the actual training.

Here is your Timetable for now. Straight from Russia. Train every day
any time of the day you wish.

	Sets x Reps	Male	Female
Swings	5 x 10 (In total)	24 kg	16 kg
Get-Ups	5 x 1 (for each arm)	16 kg	8 kg

What is a Swing? What is a Get-Up? Read on to find out.

Between different reps, you should rest until you can talk aga
without being out breath. In this resting period, do nothing. Simp
stand or walk around while breathing.

When the exercises become too easy, you will want to progress on
a different timetable. The moves will largely be the same. Kettlebe
are simple. But they will make you strong incredibly FAST.

So, if you want to find additional plans, I recommend buying furth
books on the subject.

Warming up for Kettlebell exercises

Like I said before, you want your warmups to be specific to yo
strength training. The one I designed for Tabata training is not custo
made for Kettlebells, so the Russians devised their own plan.

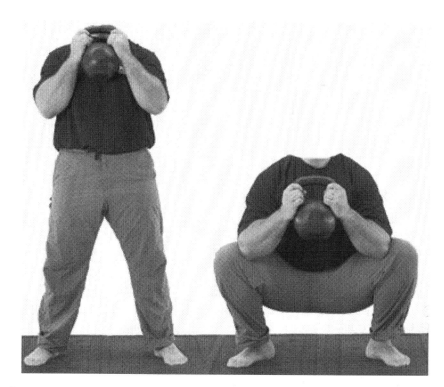

e first warmup exercise is the **Prying Goblin Squat**. It aims to open
ur hips up so that you can effectively perform later movements.

art by standing with your toes slightly outwards, with feet slightly
ɔre than shoulder-width apart. You should firmly hold on to the
ttlebell with both hands on either side of the handle.

gin to slowly push your knees outwards and sit back – not directly
wnwards – as you assume the final squat position. Make sure that
ur back is straight and that your buttocks are as low as you can get
ɘm. Your toes are still facing outwards and your feet lie flat.

w feel the weight of the Kettlebell pushing your arms and elbows
ainst your legs. The force will apply a decent stretch.

wever, to fully widen your pelvis, you must also start prying. You do
s by changing the force you apply to either leg with your elbows.
st lean onto your right leg, and then your left leg, continuing to
ernate so as to slowly but surely open your hips to a greater extent.

Do not allow your back to arch, or your arms to drop. When you have sufficiently widened your hips, stand up the same way you got into the squat. Do not let your body be misaligned and rise slowly to demonstrate a greater level of control.

The next stretch is the **Hip Bridge**, as seen earlier in the book.

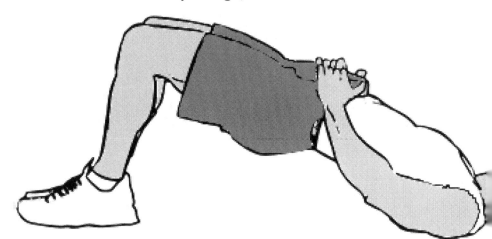

However, this time keep your knees tight together and remember to extend your hips as opposed to arching your lower back. Once fully extended, hold the position for three full seconds, and then slowly move your hips back to the ground and relax. Repeat five times.

The next warmup exercise is the **Halo**.

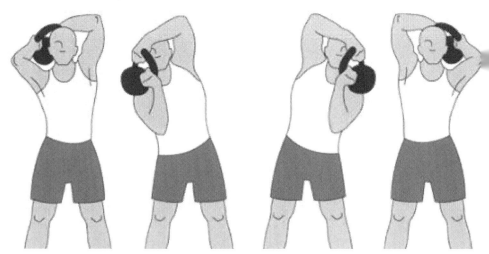

asp the Kettlebell from either sides of its handle and hold it close to ur chest. Make sure your legs form a solid base. Circle the Kettlebell er your head and back to your chest. Repeat this five times circling the left, and five times circling to the right.

total, you want to perform the Prying Goblin Squad, Hip Bridge, and lo and then **repeat all this a further two times**.

ree Fundamental Kettlebell Exercises

ere were only two Kettlebell exercises in the timetable given earlier. wever, you want to first verify whether you can handle the ttlebell safely to begin with. That is why I will first get you to do a uple of deadlifts first.

e **deadlift** looks deceptively simple, but will teach you a basic nciple that you will use in more advanced moves – the hip hinge.

rt with the Kettlebell between your feet. Point your feet less than ty-five degrees outwards, with your legs kept straight. As you bend er to reach for the Kettlebell, try to keep your shins vertical.

re is the critical part. Do not bend over using your lower back.

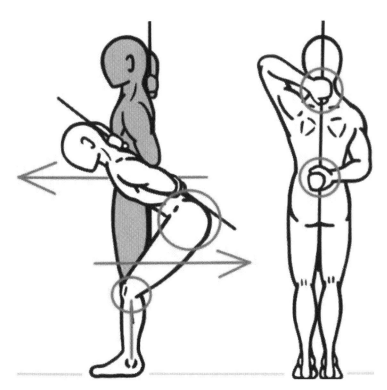

Instead, focus on the opening of your hips and use this as a lever. I
were to put a meter ruler on your back while in this position, it woul
lie flat.

As you bend down, make sure to maintain a straight back and straigh
neck. It is crucial that you look ahead and not down, since you do no
want to put too much stress on your neck when lifting.

Press your shoulders down — away from the head — but keep then
above your pelvis. In turn, your pelvis should be above your knee
Keep your bodyweight centred more towards your heels and mak
sure you have a firm grasp of the Kettlebell.

Before you get ready to stand up, relax your armpits and do not hol
on to the handle too tightly. Then, straighten your body upward.
using your glutes. Your shoulders should rise faster than your pelvi
working together as one life how your body would move in a jump.

the final standing position, tighten all your muscles as though you
e a hard board. Your abdominal muscles, glutes, legs and back
iould all be kept tight. That was one deadlift.

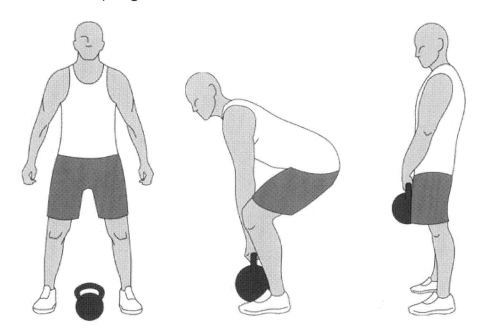

ice you can perform the deadlift with good technique and balance,
 per the picture, you are ready for the first technique featured in
ur timetable.

e **Swing** strengthens and heals your body at the same time.

re is the two-arm variety.

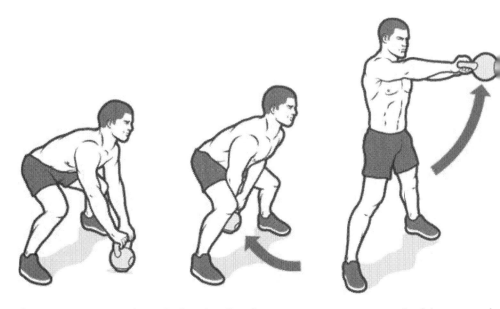

The one-arm variety is basically the same except you hold on to th
Kettlebell with one arm, and then let the other arm swing naturall
The unoccupied arm will act as a counterbalance. But because of th
nature of this book, I will only cover the two-arm variety here.

Begin by placing the Kettlebell in front of you. Get into the hip-hing
position, previously discussed, then hold on to the Kettlebell with
firm grasp. Using your arms, actively throw the bell backward
through your legs – while keeping a hold of it obviously. You shou
feel your forearms pressing tightly against your legs. In this positio
let the bell pendulum forwards loosely.

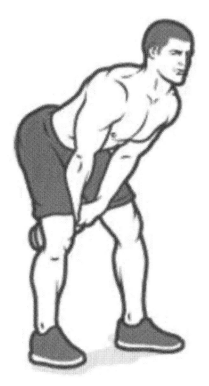

at is the key to this exercise, you push the bell back through your
s using your arms, but do <u>not</u> use your arms or shoulders to swing
e Kettlebell forwards.

ce you have let it pendulum a couple of times, use your hips to
ɔlosively swing the Kettlebell forwards.

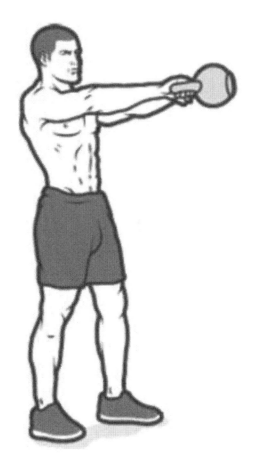

Do not swing the Kettlebell higher than your chin. You want to kee
good control of it and maintain your balance throughout.

Remember, it is your hips that propelled the bell forwards – not yo
arms swinging it upwards.

At the top, do not learn backwards. Brace your abdominal muscle
and let your glutes do the work. You do not want your back involved

For better performance, exhale at the top. I typically like to grunt as
release of energy, and some martial artists prefer to shout *ha!*

One it has reached the top, you will feel it float for a brief moment
mid-air. Then let your arms gradually guide it downwards and throu
your legs, thus completing a single repetition of the swing.

he third and final fundamental Kettlebell exercise is the **Get-Up**. This xercise builds up the torso. For any of you reading this book purely ɔ have an attractive body, here is your chance.

ɔ become a professional strongman, one approach to take is to chieve mastery of the Get-Up. By starting small and gradually orking up to seventy or a hundred pound weights, one can achieve credible levels of strength.

ere is the complete Turkish Get-Up.

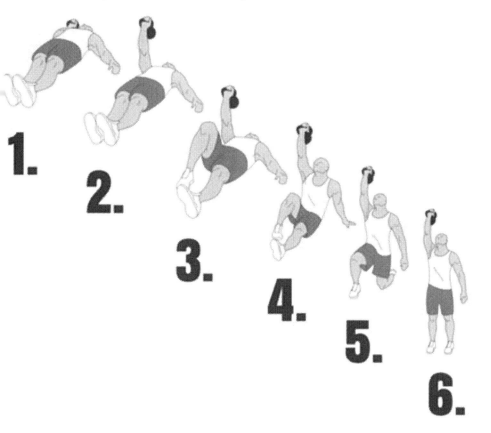

fore you try it with a Kettlebell, just go through the actions with an ɪpty hand. Learn to flow from one step to the other. Once you have mpleted all the six steps, do them in reverse to get back to the start sition so that you can start again.

Try not to rush to the heavy weights just yet. Even a shoe will do a your weight to begin with.

The details of the Turkish Get-Up are critical. You want to perform as efficiently as possible. The details of the Get-Up are very involve and written in full at the end of the chapter. However, to learn properly, you must practice it and watch videos of other people doin it online. That is the best way to learn it safely for yourself and hel you to get strong FAST.

If you find your Get-Ups becoming weak and shaky, only perfor segments of the full exercise. Stop at the part of the lift where you st feel in full control over your body. If you can do the Get-Up in slov motion then you can be sure that you are in control of your body.

The Get-Up is a characteristic slow lift whereas the Swing is a typic quick lift. Together, they cover all aspects of Strength.

Eventually, if you stick with it, you will work up to the Human Turkis Get-Up. You will slowly increase the weight of the Kettlebell that yc perform the Turkish Get-Up with. I was too excited to try it out ar lifted my girlfriend into the air only to let go too early... and have h land on the mattress. Phew.

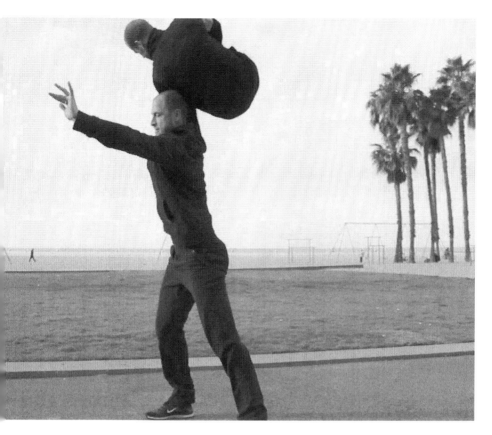

vill close this chapter with a strong image of a strong man. Being able
lift a person with one arm sure sounds strong to me.

hat's amazing is **it does not take years to master**.

ick to it for a few months, and you too **will** get strong FAST.

***

Details of the Turkish Get-Up

 down flat on the floor, with the Kettlebell next to your strong arm
rom here on, this is assumed to be your right hand. Roll to your right
e and hold on to the Kettlebell with both arms. Then roll on your
ck and grasp it only with your right hand. Lift this weight up,
suring your elbow is locked out and that your arm is held fully
rtical. Keep your right arm extended for the rest of the exercise.

[Note: you must roll. Simply lifting the Kettlebell from your side wi[ll]
injure your shoulder.]

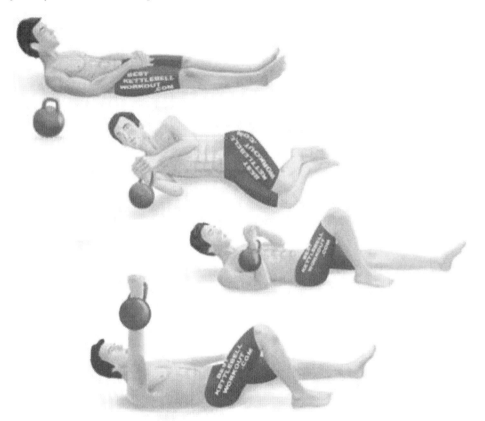

Plant your right foot firmly on the ground, effectively bending yo[ur]
knee and raising your hips. Lift your right shoulder off the floor, a[nd]
set yourself up on your elbow. Then plant yourself onto your hand ▶
pushing off the elbow. Your hand should be placed behind your hea[d]
so as to create a strong triangular structure of support.

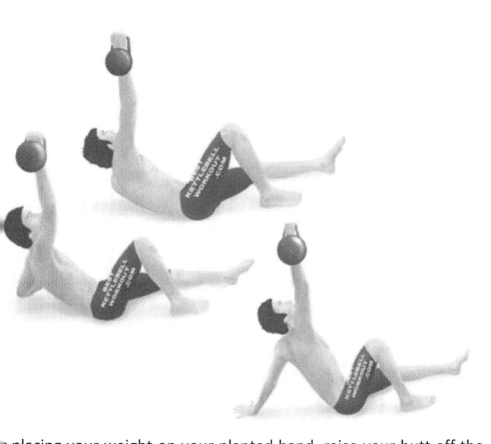

placing your weight on your planted hand, raise your butt off the
or and sweep your left leg through. The heel of your left leg will be
ectly beneath your butt, whereas the left knee will be forty-five
grees to your left. Push yourself upwards **using your back leg**, and
eferably on your toes. This is important. A lot of people push
emselves off their front leg. Using your back leg is much more
werful.

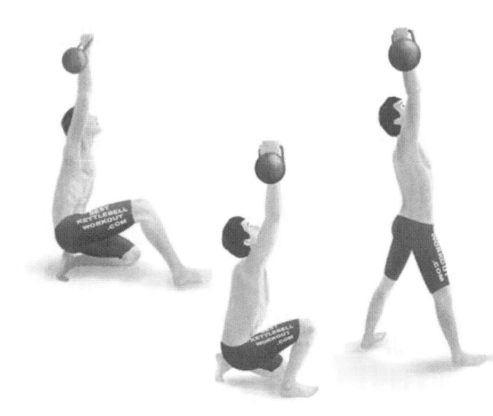

Once complete, you run the whole exercise in reverse to get back t
your starting position. The first few times you try this, do it with yo
first or a shoe on your fist. Only once you can perform the who
exercise smoothly and almost **effortlessly**, do you pick up th
Kettlebell and begin to get strong FAST.

Closing Words

I gave you five secrets. It is up to you which secret you want to use in your life – if any. Simply holding the Superman Pose changed my life. In fact, it was the first secret I learnt. Maybe you have already started to breathe like Wim Hof. Or perhaps you have bought yourself some kettlebells.

So, did I keep my promise? Depends on whether you kept your end of the bargain. It is time for you to go right now and become strong FAST.

Eat great food.

Get rid of your bad habits and conquer your true will.

Breathe in all the oxygen your body wants.

Shower yourself in pure coldness.

Train for a few minutes every day.

I'm sure you can visualise the new you right now.

Now remember what you learnt from me and change your life.

Three months. That is your challenge.

Get strong FAST!

Good Luck!

15319608R00060

Printed in Great Britain
by Amazon